DAILY EXERCISE INTEGRATION

DYNAMIC FITNESS ROUTINES, EXERCISE RECOVERY METHODS, AND MORE

FUNCTIONAL HEALTH SERIES

SAM FURY

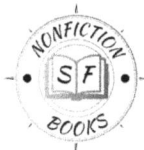

WARNINGS AND DISCLAIMERS

The information in this publication is made public for reference only.

Neither the author, publisher, nor anyone else involved in the production of this publication is responsible for how the reader uses the information or the result of his/her actions.

Nothing presented is medical advice. Implement anything you learn at your own risk. If in doubt, please consult a medical professional.

CONTENTS

All books in the Functional Health Series are transcriptions of masterclasses from within our members area.

As a member, you will get full access to all these masterclasses in eBook and audio format and a whole lot more at no extra cost.

Get 30 days access for just $1!

www.longevitypillars.com

INTRODUCTION

Inside this guide, you will discover everything you need to integrate adaptable and effective exercise habits into your daily life. Written for individuals at all fitness levels, this guide aims to make exercise a natural and evolving part of your lifestyle.

At its core is the principle of dynamic fitness, an approach that emphasizes flexibility in your fitness regime. This approach involves creating a routine that evolves with your changing needs, goals, and lifestyle, ensuring that your exercise remains effective, enjoyable, and aligned with your personal growth. Whether you are just beginning your fitness journey or looking to revamp your current routine, this dynamic fitness approach is designed to help a broad audience develop an adaptable exercise plan that is unique to each individual's situation.

Your journey starts with understanding your motivation and setting realistic fitness goals. These steps are foundational in creating a dynamic fitness routine that helps you tailor your exercise regime to your evolving life and goals. This versatile mindset is crucial for keeping your workouts relevant and engaging over time.

We will dive into critical components of fitness other than exercise: nutrition, hydration, and sleep. These elements are not fluff, but rather essential for supporting your exercise routine. Here, you will learn practical advice on optimizing them.

Arm yourself with knowledge of injury prevention, management, and recovery, which are vital to maintaining long term workout plans. This book will equip you with the knowledge to improve your fitness routine while nurturing your body.

It's important to be aware of how your changing fitness level and personal circumstances should lead to adjustments in your fitness program. Strength training and cardiovascular conditioning exercises must be frequently evaluated, and we will show how you can switch between different exercise types and difficulty levels in order to keep your workout fresh and challenging.

Flexibility and balance, often overlooked in more rigid programs, are critical for a well-rounded fitness routine. You will learn how to incorporate these elements into your personal training program, thus enhancing your overall fitness and reducing the risk of injury, all while adapting to the shifts in your daily life.

You will also learn about active recovery techniques, which are methods that help your body recover and prepare for future workouts.

Personalizing your fitness journey is the culmination of this guide. Recognizing that each individual's body, goals, and life situations are unique, you'll gain insights into creating a routine that is as adaptable and flexible as life itself, including an outline into my own fitness routine, which you can use for yourself or adapt as needed.

This is not just a guide to exercising, but a comprehensive blueprint for weaving a flexible, responsive, and effective fitness regime into the fabric of your everyday life. Let's get started!

FITNESS GOALS AND MOTIVATION

Setting fitness goals and staying motivated are essential aspects of integrating exercise into your life. Just like finding the right path on a road trip or keeping track of your progress along the way, these elements help ensure you reach your destination. In this chapter, we will explore the key factors that drive and help you maintain your motivation for fitness, from identifying your 'why' to setting SMART goals, tracking your progress, and harnessing motivation boosters. Whether you're starting your fitness journey or looking to revitalize your routine, understanding these principles will be your roadmap to success.

Finding Your Why

"Finding Your Why" is about identifying the core reason behind achieving whatever it is you want to achieve. In this case, it's about delving deep into your personal motivations and understanding what will truly drive you to maintain a fitness regimen. This "why" is the foundation your fitness journey is built on, and it serves as a powerful motivator, especially during times when your dedication is tested.

When you find your "why," your fitness dream becomes more than just a goal; it transforms into a personal mission. This could be as specific as wanting to improve your health to be active with your children or as broad as seeking overall well-being. For many, their 'why' is tied to long-term health benefits. Understanding that regular exercise can prevent or manage health issues like hypertension, heart disease, or diabetes provides a strong incentive to stay active.

Your "why" might also be rooted in mental health benefits. Regular physical activity is known to alleviate symptoms of depression and anxiety. For those struggling with mental health challenges, exercise can become a crucial part of their coping strategy, providing a natural and effective way to boost mood and mental clarity.

For some, their "why" is about physical appearance and self-esteem. The desire to feel confident in one's own skin can be a compelling motivator. This often involves setting specific appearance-based goals, like reaching a certain weight or body composition, which can provide a clear and measurable target to work toward.

In many cases, the "why" is associated with social factors. Whether it's the camaraderie of a sports team, the community in a fitness class, or even an online fitness group, the social aspect of exercise can be a strong motivator. For these individuals, their fitness journey is also a social journey, providing a sense of belonging and mutual support.

The key to "Finding Your Why" is introspection. It requires taking time to reflect on what really matters to you, what you value, and what you hope to achieve through your fitness journey. It's a personal exploration that can lead to a deeper understanding of your motivations, which in turn makes your fitness goals more meaningful and attainable.

Remember, your "why" is unique to you and may differ from someone else's. It's not about comparing motivations but about understanding what drives you personally. Once you've identified your "why," it serves as a constant reminder and source of inspiration that keeps you focused and committed, especially on days when motivation is low.

Assessing Your Current Fitness Level

Assessing your current fitness level is a crucial first step in your fitness journey, like taking a snapshot of your current health so that you can plan your path forward. This process involves understanding your strengths, weaknesses, and areas that need improvement. Think of it like knowing your location before embarking on a road trip; it's essential for charting your route to your destination.

Self-assessment gives you a clear starting point. By evaluating your strength, endurance, flexibility, and other fitness components, you gain a realistic picture of your physical capabilities. This knowledge acts as a guide that directs you toward your goals.

Setting realistic goals prevents you from overestimating your fitness level—a danger in which you would risk aiming for unachievable objectives, leading to frustration or injury. Conversely, underestimating your abilities might result in insufficient challenges. Self-assessment ensures your fitness goals are appropriate and achievable.

Knowing your starting point and desired endpoint can spark determination, allowing self-assessment to fuel your motivation, much like anticipating a beautiful beach at the end of a road trip. A clear vision of your potential improvement will keep you committed and motivated.

To use the road trip analogy again, self-assessment allows you to track your progress like when you check your GPS during a road trip. Regular fitness assessments enable you to see how far you've come, adjust your goals, celebrate achievements, and focus on areas needing more attention.

An integral part of assessing your fitness is conducting a health check—like inspecting your car before a long journey. This check includes measuring vital signs like blood pressure and heart rate, evaluating body composition through the body mass index (BMI) and body measurements, and assessing cardiovascular fitness through exercises like walking or jogging. It's also important to consider any existing health conditions or injuries and consult with healthcare professionals as needed.

A physical fitness assessment extends beyond basic health checks, diving deeper into your physical health and abilities. This comprehensive evaluation includes measuring strength, endurance, flexibility, and assessing skills like agility, balance, and coordination. It also involves evaluating body composition to set realistic weight-related goals and track changes over time.

Lastly, setting baseline measurements is vital. These measurements, including weight, body measurements, and body composition, serve as a reference point to track progress and determine if you're moving closer to your goals. Knowing these numbers provides a clear picture of your physical state, aids in goal setting, motivates progress, and guides personalized fitness planning.

In summary, assessing your fitness level is like setting your GPS for a road trip. It establishes a starting point, helps set realistic goals, fuels motivation, allows for progress tracking, and includes health checks and physical fitness assessments to tailor your journey to your specific needs. So, before you embark on your own fitness adventure, you'll need to evaluate your fitness level and use that knowledge to develop the best route.

Setting SMART Fitness Goals

In setting fitness goals, the SMART framework guides you to create goals that are Specific, Measurable, Achievable, Relevant, and Time-Bound.

- Specific: It's vital to clearly define your fitness objectives. Rather than vague goals like "I want to get fit," opt for specific targets such as "I want to increase my upper body strength by being able to do ten push-ups without resting." This approach not only identifies the area of focus but also sets a clear target, making your path forward more defined.
- Measurable: Make sure your goals allow you to track your progress. For example, instead of a broad goal like "improving cardiovascular fitness," a measurable goal would be "running five kilometers without stopping within three months." This quantifiable aspect lets you see your improvements over time and helps in maintaining motivation.
- Achievable: It's important to consider your current fitness level, available resources, and time constraints in order to set realistic targets. For instance, if new to running, a more achievable goal might be completing a 5K race rather than

a marathon. Smaller, incremental goals are not only more attainable but also build confidence and motivation.

- Relevant: Your fitness activities should align with your overall aspirations. If your primary aim is to enhance cardiovascular health, relevant goals would include increasing your daily step count or engaging in regular cardio workouts. These goals should be meaningful to you and fit within your broader fitness plan.
- Time-Bound: It's important to be able to see the finish line! Time-bound goals involve setting specific deadlines. A goal like "losing ten pounds in three months" provides a clear timeframe, which encourages consistent effort and helps you monitor your progress.

It's also crucial to distinguish between long-term and short-term goals. Long-term goals are your ultimate fitness aspirations, while short-term goals are the manageable steps you take towards achieving these larger objectives. Balancing both is key to maintaining motivation and staying on track.

Breaking down large goals into smaller, manageable steps is another effective strategy. This approach makes daunting goals feel more achievable and allows you to track your progress. If setbacks occur, these smaller milestones make it easier to adjust your plan without losing sight of the ultimate goal.

Lastly, incorporating flexibility into your SMART goals is essential. Life is unpredictable, and your fitness plan should be adaptable. Set both outcome goals (like losing weight) and process goals (performing specific daily or weekly actions). Be ready to modify these goals as circumstances change and be forgiving of setbacks. Flexibility in your approach ensures that you stay motivated and committed to your fitness journey even when challenges arise.

Tracking Progress

Tracking progress is key to achieving fitness goals and staying motivated. Like a map on a road trip, it keeps you on course, preventing you from becoming lost or demotivated. Seeing tangible improvements like milestones will boost your motivation by providing evidence of your achievements.

Monitoring progress also allows for adjustments to your fitness routine by helping identify effective strategies and areas that need change like workout adjustments, diet modifications, or new goals. This adaptability is crucial for long-term success.

Recording achievements and setbacks also acts like a personal fitness diary because it promotes accountability with yourself. This can be a powerful motivator, especially during challenging times. Additionally, fitness tracking enhances your self-awareness of your journey. You can look back through your entries in order to understand your body's response to exercises and diets as well as inform decisions for a tailored fitness plan.

But what should you track? Focus on aspects that match your specific fitness goals. Physical changes like weight, body measurements, and body fat percentage offer a clear picture of your body's response to your routine. But remember these numbers are just part of the overall health picture!

Workout performance, including exercises, sets, reps, and weight lifted, shows progress in strength and endurance. Cardiovascular fitness, tracked through activities like running or swimming, is vital for overall health and stamina. Flexibility and mobility, though less quantifiable, are crucial for injury prevention and overall fitness.

But don't forget that health involves more than just physical exercise! Nutrition tracking is another useful habit–a food diary is a great method for this–because it helps ensure that you're properly fueled for your goals, whether that's weight loss, muscle gain, or physical performance. Additionally, tracking your mood and motivation can provide insights into your mental and emotional health, which is a good reminder that fitness is not just about the body.

Technology has simplified fitness tracking, offering tools like fitness apps, wearable devices, and virtual platforms. Apps like MyFitnessPal and Fitbit log workouts and food intake, while wearables monitor steps, heart rate, and sleep quality. On top of that, specialized gadgets cater to specific activities, like GPS watches for runners. Virtual fitness platforms provide workout classes and progress tracking, making it easy to follow routines at home. Technology can even help you find other people to help you on your fitness journey! Social media and online communities offer accountability and support.

Communities can help with one of the biggest obstacles to exercise plans: plateaus. Encountering plateaus is common, and adapting to them is key to continued progress. Changing workout routines, re-evaluating nutrition, focusing on recovery and rest, setting realistic goals, and seeking professional guidance can help overcome these periods of stagnation.

Recognizing that goals should be adjustable is essential, as life is dynamic. Adjust your goals to remain realistic, cater to new challenges, and continue challenging yourself. If one month is particularly busy for you, evaluate your calendar to see what a more realistic exercise schedule might be while you navigate this busy period in life. Or perhaps you twisted your ankle on uneven ground and now you need to let it rest for a few days. Adapt your plan to account for your changing priorities and to respond to your body's changing needs. This flexibility prevents burnout and injury, allowing you to maintain a sustainable fitness routine.

In summary, progress tracking is vital for fitness because it provides motivation, allows for adjustments, and enhances self-awareness. Choosing what to track should align with personal goals, and technology can aid in this process. As you continue to improve, you should adapt to plateaus and adjust goals as needed to ensure a sustainable and effective fitness journey.

Motivation Boosters

Visualizing success is a potent tool for enhancing motivation in achieving fitness goals. This technique involves creating vivid mental images of your desired outcomes, like running a marathon or fitting into that pair of jeans that has been sitting in the back of your closet for the past five years. These images serve as a mental roadmap, guiding and motivating you throughout your fitness journey.

Not only does visualizing success help in staying focused, but it also aids in overcoming obstacles. Recalling these images during challenging times can reinforce your determination and remind you of the rewards awaiting you. Conveniently, this practice can be done anywhere, helping you stay connected to your goals.

Rewards and incentives can provide something positive in return for adhering to your workout routine or making healthy choices. Some options are treats, gifts, or recognition of achievements. By creating a sense of anticipation and excitement, rewards acknowledge your hard work and dedication, boosting self-esteem. Selecting meaningful rewards—such as new workout gear instead of food-related treats—and setting incremental milestones can be highly effective.

Variety is the spice of life and exercise plans. Monotony leads to boredom, so introducing different types of exercises or changing your workout's intensity and structure keeps your routine fresh and engaging. This approach not only prevents overuse injuries but also aids in breaking through progress plateaus, making exercise more enjoyable and mentally stimulating.

Music is a way to keep you going as you work through your fitness routine. It enhances your mood, distracts you from fatigue, and you can synchronize it with your movements, making workouts feel smoother and more engaging. Personal preferences in music play a significant role—a familiar playlist can signal to your brain that it's time to exercise, which can help you get in the workout mood.

If you're looking to add excitement and purpose to your workouts, competition and challenges could be an excellent fitness approach!

Competing against yourself or others, whether through personal goals or group activities, ignites a competitive spirit. This not only pushes you to improve but also fosters a sense of community, providing support and accountability.

In summary, visualizing success, rewarding accomplishments, varying workouts, listening to music, and competing with others are all effective strategies to boost motivation on your fitness journey. Each element adds a unique dimension to staying motivated and achieving your fitness goals.

Motivation Though Others

Even if you're not feeling competitive, adding a social element to your fitness journey can be a powerful motivator. It's helpful to surround yourself with like-minded individuals, such as training partners or participating in group classes. When you have someone by your side, you're more likely to stay committed and accountable to your fitness routine.

Training partners can provide that extra push you need during your workouts. Whether it's a friend, family member, or even a colleague, an exercise companion can make the process more enjoyable and inspiring. Sharing the sweat and effort can create a sense of camaraderie, making it easier to stick to your fitness goals.

Group classes are another fantastic option for finding motivation through others. These classes bring together individuals with similar objectives and are led by an instructor. Being part of a group not only adds a social aspect to your workouts but also creates a sense of belonging and friendly competition. The energy and encourage- ment from fellow participants can help you stay motivated and committed to your fitness journey.

You could even find classmates that could act as an accountability partner! Accountability partners are there to hold you responsible for your actions and decisions regarding your fitness goals. It could be a friend, family member, or even someone you meet at the gym.

Knowing that someone is checking in on your progress can keep you on track and motivated to push forward.

In addition to training partners and group classes, coaches and mentors can be instrumental in boosting your motivation. Coaches have the knowledge and experience to provide personalized guidance and support. They will set realistic goals, track your progress, and offer expert advice, which can be incredibly motivating. Mentors, on the other hand, are individuals who have already achieved the fitness goals you're striving for. Their success stories and guidance can serve as a powerful source of inspiration, helping you believe in your own potential.

Takeaways

Finding motivation through others can be a game-changer in your fitness journey. The support, camaraderie, and accountability they provide can help you stay motivated and committed to your fitness goals, making the path to a healthier lifestyle more enjoyable and achievable.

Staying motivated on your fitness journey is like having a reliable co-pilot on a road trip. Motivation is what keeps you on track, helps you navigate through challenges, and ultimately guides you towards your destination: a healthier and fitter version of yourself. By finding your "why," setting SMART goals, tracking your progress, and leveraging motivation boosters or support from others, you can ensure a smooth and rewarding fitness journey. Remember, it's not just about reaching your fitness goals; it's about enjoying the ride and the transformation it brings to your life.

INTEGRATING EXERCISE INTO YOUR LIFE

Integrating exercise into your daily life is essential for nurturing both physical and mental health. This chapter delves into the practical aspects of making exercise an integral and enjoyable part of your routine. From embracing small, consistent steps to involving your social circle, it offers insights into establishing a sustainable fitness habit. Balancing exercise with life's demands isn't just about scheduling; it's about creating a lifestyle that values health as a cornerstone. Whether it's through active commuting, workplace fitness, or shared activities with loved ones, this chapter guides you in weaving exercise seamlessly into the fabric of your daily life.

Increasing Daily Movement

The key to success in almost all things in life lies in consistency, and things are no different here. Consistency in exercise means adhering to a regular routine and transforming physical activity into a habitual part of your life. You establish a routine by making exercise a priority and a natural part of daily life, whether through a morning jog or an evening swim. Regular exercise improves fitness levels as the body adapts to physical demands, becoming stronger and more efficient, much like learning a skill or language.

A steady exercise routine can additionally improve mental health, for example by reducing stress and depression, and can boost your mood by releasing endorphins. Consistent daily exercise also allows for tracking progress and making adjustments, which are crucial for long-term success. Establishing a workout routine is vital for achieving specific fitness goals like weight loss or muscle building.

To create a lifelong exercise habit, start with small, manageable goals that will help you avoid burnout. Begin with simple activities like a 15-minute daily walk or a quick home workout and maintain a regular schedule to make these habits stick. You can then gradually increase intensity as your confidence and endurance increase.

Finding enjoyable activities is also crucial. Engaging in exercises you love, like dancing or swimming, makes it more likely you'll stick with it. It's worth repeating: Consistency is the cornerstone of success! Treat exercise like any other important activity in your life.

Enjoyable, consistent exercise is even easier if you are held accountable for your exercise habits in some way. Partner with a person who shares your fitness goals for mutual motivation. If you can't find an exercise partner, there are accountability alternatives. Tracking progress, whether through a journal or an app, can help you maintain focus, and it's important to be patient and forgiving with yourself. Understand that building a lifelong habit takes time and occasional setbacks are normal.

Involving your family and friends in your exercise journey can be incredibly beneficial! Group activities like biking or hiking not only promote fitness but also strengthen relationships. Joining group fitness classes or sports leagues adds a social element, making exercise more enjoyable. Setting shared goals or challenges can also boost motivation.

Active commuting, like walking or cycling to work, is another opportunity to integrate exercise into your daily routine. It's beneficial for the environment and your health and wallet. If you commute over a long distance, you could consider combining active commuting with public transportation.

Finally, incorporating exercise into your workplace can significantly increase your daily movement. Not sure how to do so? Take active breaks, use a standing desk, or hold walking meetings. You could also utilize any fitness facilities provided by your employer, consider active commuting, and encourage a culture of physical activity among colleagues.

Balancing Exercise With Other Life Commitments

Integrating exercise into your existing schedule may seem difficult at the start, but it is one of the key steps toward an active lifestyle. And, to be honest, it isn't actually that hard to do. In fact, once you start, you may wonder how you lived without it!

Fitting exercise into your daily routine makes it less of a chore and more of a habit. Consider waking up earlier for a morning workout or using lunch breaks for a brisk walk.

However, don't wake up too early! Prioritizing rest and recovery is just as important. Overworking yourself without adequate rest can lead to burnout and negatively impact your health, so make sure you include rest days in your routine and ensure you get sufficient sleep.

Time management is vital for balancing exercise and other commitments. Create a daily or weekly schedule to allocate specific times for exercise, treating that time as important as any other commitment. If you prefer a weekly task list rather than an hour-by-hour calendar, then prioritize exercise and make sure that it is high on your list. What if time is of the essence? Consider multitasking, like exercising during a meeting that doesn't require your physical presence, and learn to say no to overcommitting. If you need help developing and staying on schedule, technology and apps can aid in scheduling workouts and tracking progress.

That being said, keep in mind that it's good to remain flexible and be adaptable if unexpected events arise. Life is dynamic, with events like new jobs, parenthood, or illness necessitating adjustments to your exercise routine. Reassess priorities during these times and communicate your needs to those around you. Be kind to yourself—always remember that it's okay to modify your routine. Explore new exercise options that fit your current situation and revisit your goals while adjusting them as needed.

The path to a healthier life is not just about rigorous routines; it's about making exercise a natural and enjoyable part of your everyday existence. Embrace the journey, celebrate the small victories, and let each step take you closer to a life where health and happiness are in harmony.

Nutrition, Hydration, and Sleep

Nutrition, hydration, and sleep all play crucial roles in determining the effectiveness of exercise. Proper nutrition ensures that your body has the necessary fuel to perform at its best by providing energy for workouts and aiding in muscle recovery afterward.

Hydration is equally vital, as dehydration can lead to decreased performance, fatigue, and an increased risk of injury. Staying adequately hydrated helps regulate body temperature and maintains essential bodily functions during exercise.

As far as sufficient sleep is concerned, it is essential for muscle recovery, hormone regulation, and overall physical and mental well-being. Lack of sleep can impair cognitive function, reduce motivation to exercise, and hinder the body's ability to repair and adapt to the stresses of physical activity.

In this section, we will not be delving deep into each of those subjects. Instead, I will give you the main actionable steps you can apply, and, if you want more information, you can refer to the other books in the Functional Health Series that are dedicated to each of those topics.

Nutrition and Hydration

Modern nutrition advice can be very overwhelming, and there is a lot of conflicting information out there. With new science and fad theories emerging all the time, it is hard to know what to follow. However, there are fundamental principles that the vast majority of science-based health advocates agree on.

First of all, minimize ultra-processed foods. Ultra-processed foods are often found in brightly colored packaging with long ingredient lists. They typically contain high levels of added sugars, unhealthy fats, and artificial additives. Instead, prioritize fresh foods like fruits, vegetables, and lean proteins.

Strive to consume approximately one gram of protein per pound of your target body weight, just as a general guideline. Lean protein sources are best, such as lean meats, fish, tofu, eggs, and legumes.

You should also aim to fill at least half of your plate with freshly grown food. Don't worry, fruit counts here as well, not just vegetables. The more variety, the better; however, if you find it challenging to eat vegetables, start by choosing the ones you like and gradually branch out to others.

As for what you should drink every day, you've probably heard this advice before, but it's true and worth repeating: Prioritize water as your primary beverage and make sure you drink enough of it. A good rule of thumb, as proposed by Dr. Mark Hyman, is to drink half your weight (in pounds) in ounces of water. So, if you weigh 100 pounds, you should aim to drink around 50 ounces of water a day. When in hot climates or exerting more energy, such as during exercise, you will need more water. Listening to your body is key – thirst is a natural indicator of the need for water.

Finally, don't forget to incorporate fermented foods and healthy fats into your daily diet. Fermented foods are great for your gut health and include items like kimchi, Greek yogurt, kefir, sauerkraut, and kombucha. Healthy fats include olive oil, avocado oil, fatty fish, eggs, seeds, and nuts. Of course, these lists are not exhaustive.

While the barrage of nutrition information can be daunting, adhering to these cornerstone principles of consuming whole foods, staying hydrated, and balancing your diet with a variety of proteins, fruits, vegetables, healthy fats, and fermented foods will provide a solid foundation for good health. Remember, moderation and balance are key, and making gradual changes can lead to lasting health benefits.

Sleep Hygiene

Sleep is ultra-important for overall health for a variety of reasons. When it comes to your exercise regime specifically, a good night's sleep allows your body to repair and regenerate muscle tissues, regulate hormones essential for recovery and performance, and recharge energy levels, enhancing overall physical performance and reducing the risk of injury. Sleep hygiene involves adopting habits and environmental factors conducive to healthy and restful sleep.

Here are my top tips that you can start implementing tonight, and each is cheap to implement, if not free:

- Scheduling: Establish a consistent sleep schedule. The average person needs around eight hours of sleep a night, give or take an hour. Set your bedtime to eight or nine hours before the time you need to wake up and make an effort to adhere to this schedule as consistently as possible. The more you stick to the schedule, the easier it will be to fall asleep each night!
- Avoid Stimulants: Once you've determined your bedtime, plan when to stop consuming stimulants. Stimulants come in various forms, but we'll focus on the most common ones in this brief overview:

1. Caffeine: This can impact your sleep cycle long after consumption, so it's advisable to stop caffeine intake at least eight hours before bedtime.
2. Artificial Lights: Think about all those lights emitted by your TV, computer, tablets, and phones—they also act as common stimulants. This even includes the small LEDs on your chargers! Ideally, avoid exposure to this "junk light" for at least one hour before bedtime, preferably longer.
3. Food and Drink: Consuming them too close to bedtime means that even though you're asleep, your body is still working to process the nutrients. This can disrupt your sleep quality and lead to digestive discomfort during the night.

- Environment: Ideally, your sleeping environment should be cool, dark, and quiet, with access to fresh air. If necessary, use earplugs or a white noise machine to block out noise.

To prevent light from disturbing your sleep, consider blackout curtains or an eye mask.

- Natural Light: In line with the importance of light, make an effort to get natural sunlight each day. This helps regulate your body's circadian rhythm. Ideally, aim for early morning sunlight upon waking up and late afternoon sunlight, as well.

Takeaways

By integrating physical activity into your daily routine through steps such as active commuting, workplace fitness, and social workouts, you can make significant strides towards better health. Additionally, by focusing on whole foods, adequate hydration, and establishing a healthy sleep routine, you equip your body with the necessary tools for optimal performance and recovery.

The journey to better health doesn't require intricate knowledge or expensive solutions; simple, consistent steps in the right direction are often the most effective. As you apply these principles, observe the positive changes in your fitness levels and general health, and continue to adapt and refine your approach for ongoing success.

INJURY PREVENTION, MANAGEMENT, AND RECOVERY

This chapter offers valuable insights into preventing, managing, and effectively recovering from common injuries associated with exercise. It covers a wide range of exercise-related injuries, including strains, sprains, and more complex issues such as stress fractures and tendinitis.

The primary focus is on comprehending the underlying causes, identifying symptoms, and implementing suitable measures to ensure a safe and healthy exercise regimen. Additionally, the chapter underscores the significance of maintaining proper form and technique, as well as the role of cross-training and nutrition in injury prevention and recovery. By presenting a holistic perspective, it endeavors to empower you with the knowledge necessary to protect your physical well-being throughout your fitness journey.

Understanding Common Exercise-Related Injuries

Exercise-related injuries, which can affect anyone from beginners to seasoned athletes, vary in severity and impact different body parts. Awareness of these injuries is key for effective prevention, management, and recovery.

Common Injuries and How to Avoid Them

Strains and sprains are perhaps the most common types of exercise injuries. Strains occur when your muscle or tendon tears due to overexertion or improper exercise form. Sprains, however, occur when your ligaments that connect bones stretch or tear. So, it makes sense that activities involving sudden movements or excessive force, like heavy weightlifting or quick directional changes in sports, often lead to these injuries.

Gymnastics, on the other hand, is likely to cause injuries like stress fractures, which are tiny cracks in bones caused by repetitive impact and overuse. These typically affect lower limbs and lead to pain, swelling, and difficulty with walking or running. Tendinitis, the inflammation of tendons attaching muscles to bones, similarly results from overuse or incorrect biomechanics. It causes pain, swelling, and limited motion, often in shoulders, elbows, knees, and ankles. You might expect this type of injury to be more common in sports like golf or tennis.

You should be on the lookout for some common injuries regardless of the activity. Dehydration or electrolyte imbalances can cause muscle cramps, which are sudden painful muscle contractions during or after exercise. Contusions, or bruises, often result from direct blows during physical activities that damage blood vessels under the skin, causing discoloration and localized pain.

Overtraining syndrome can occur when someone undergoes excessive training without adequate time for recovery, which can lead to fatigue, persistent muscle soreness, decreased performance, and mood disturbances. Recognizing these injuries is essential for individuals and fitness professionals to prevent injuries, ensure safe exercise, and facilitate recovery.

Common Causes of Injury

Understanding the causes of exercise-related injuries is crucial. Improper technique or form during physical activities, like lifting weights with incorrect back posture, increases injury risk. Overexertion by pushing beyond one's limits without adequate rest can lead to muscle strains or stress fractures. If you skip warm-up exercises or neglect stretching before vigorous activities, you increase the risk of strains, sprains, and muscle pulls.

Injuries can come from more than just your form–it's important to exercise with the proper equipment! Engaging in activities without adequate conditions can strain muscles, ligaments, and tendons. Using worn-out or ill-fitting athletic shoes or outdated equipment can result in injuries like plantar fasciitis or ankle sprains. Environmental conditions, such as extreme weather, can also contribute to exercise-related injuries like dehydration, heatstroke, or frostbite.

Another important risk factor for exercise-related injuries is age, even if we don't like to think about how old we are. Older individuals often have less flexible muscles and therefore recover more slowly. You're also more likely to have a history of previous injuries when you're older. Unfortunately, previous injury history increases re-injury risk due to residual weakness or altered movement patterns. So, when considering your susceptibility to injuries, it's important to consider your body's age and past history along with your physical fitness level, warm-up and cool-down routines, biomechanics or alignment, and amount of exercise—there is such a thing as too much!

Recognizing the warning signs of exercise-related injuries is crucial. Persistent pain during or after exercise, swelling, decreased range of motion, weakness or instability in muscles or joints, changes in exercise form or technique, and unusual sensations or noises during exercise should prompt immediate attention to prevent further problems. For example, if you hear a pop while lifting something heavy, even if you don't feel any pain, you should get it checked out.

Warm-Up and Cool-Down

Warming up and cooling down play critical roles in any physical activity routine because they significantly reduce the risk of injuries. Beginning with a warm-up is essential, as it prepares your muscles and joints for strenuous activity by gradually increasing your heart rate and blood flow. This process enhances muscle flexibility and readies your body for action, effectively lowering the likelihood of strains or tears. Additionally, warming up sharpens your coordination and reaction time, making you more alert and better equipped to handle the demands of your activity. Skipping this crucial step can leave your body unprepared and increase the risk of sprains or more severe injuries.

Transitioning to the cooling down phase is just as important as warming up. It aids your body in smoothly returning to its resting state, preventing sudden drops in heart rate that can lead to dizziness. Continuing to move during the cooling down phase also helps eliminate waste products such as lactic acid from your muscles, reducing post-exercise soreness and stiffness, which is especially vital for recovery after intense physical activity.

So, what is a good warm up? Cardiovascular warm-ups are specifically designed to target your heart and circulatory system. Activities like brisk walking, jogging, or cycling before your main exercise allow you to gradually increase your heart and breathing rates. This prepares your muscles by providing them with essential nutrients and oxygen, rendering them pliable and reducing the risk of injuries. Warm-ups provide good mental preparation, as well! They help you be mentally ready for exercise by enhancing your focus and concentration.

Understanding the difference between dynamic and static stretching is key. Dynamic stretching, which involves active movements, is ideal during a warm-up. It not only increases blood flow but also prepares your body for specific movements, reducing the risk of injury. On the other hand, static stretching, where you hold a position, is best reserved for the cooling down phase. It relaxes and elongates muscles, improving flexibility and promoting recovery.

Another important aspect of a comprehensive warm-up is targeted muscle activation. This technique involves engaging specific muscle groups that are relevant to your activity. For instance, exercises like leg swings or lunges activate leg muscles when preparing for running. This enhances coordination and balance, further reducing the risk of strains or injuries.

And don't forget cool downs! Gradually reducing the intensity of your activity lowers your heart and breathing rates safely. Stretching during this phase focuses on enhancing flexibility and relieving muscle tension. How so? It helps relax your muscles, increase blood flow, and eliminate exercise byproducts like lactic acid. Incorporating stretching into your cool-down routine contributes to long-term muscle and joint health, further reducing the risk of injuries.

Form, Technique, and Rest

Preventing, managing, and recovering from injuries in physical activities largely hinges on the importance of proper form and technique. Proper form, the correct way of performing exercises or movements, is crucial for avoiding unnecessary stress on the body. For instance, incorrect posture during weight lifting or squats can lead to muscle, joint, or back strains, impeding your fitness journey and daily life.

Maintaining proper form is not only vital for injury prevention but also for ensuring you target the intended muscles effectively during workouts. This balanced muscle development prevents overuse injuries and enhances overall strength and fitness. Proper form also boosts performance, allowing for heavier lifts, faster runs, and better sport-specific skills.

Another aspect to consider is avoiding common exercise mistakes. Rushing through exercises without proper movement can strain muscles and joints. Lifting weights that are too heavy too soon, skipping warm-ups and cool-downs, overtraining, and neglecting proper nutrition and hydration can all hinder progress and increase injury risks.

Technique and intensity in exercise are interconnected. Technique involves proper body alignment and movement sequence, minimizing injury risks and ensuring effective muscle engagement. Intensity, the level of effort in workouts, is crucial for progress. However, focusing solely on intensity can compromise form and lead to injuries. A successful fitness journey involves starting with proper technique and gradually increasing intensity.

Lastly, finding the right balance between workout intensity and rest is critical in injury prevention. Intense workouts build strength and endurance, but without adequate rest, overtraining can occur, leading to muscle strains and fatigue. Rest days are essential for muscle recovery and replenishing energy stores. Paying attention to signs of fatigue can guide you in balancing high and low-intensity workouts with necessary rest days.

Proper form, avoiding common mistakes, balancing technique with intensity, and managing workout intensity and rest are key components in injury prevention, management, and recovery in physical activities. Prioritizing these aspects ensures a safer and more effective fitness journey.

Cross-Training for Injury Prevention

Cross-training entails engaging in a diverse range of physical activities or exercises rather than exclusively focusing on a single sport or activity. This approach offers several benefits that we'll discuss now in detail.

First, let's address the overarching health benefits. The cross-training method improves agility, flexibility, and coordination, all of which are essential for injury prevention. Engaging in diverse activities makes the body more adaptable to various movements and situations, reducing the risk of injury during sports or daily activities.

Cross-training focuses on your overall fitness and strength. Engaging in a range of activities targets different muscle groups and improves your cardiovascular endurance. This well-rounded approach helps build strength in areas that you may accidentally neglect if you focus on a single activity. For example, a cyclist may incorporate strength training or yoga into their regimen to target muscles that cycling alone may not adequately engage.

If you neglect one muscle group in favor of another, this leads to muscular imbalances that can increase the risk of injury. Many individuals develop strength imbalances from their preferred sports or activities. By addressing weaker areas and promoting muscle symmetry, cross-training helps rectify these imbalances.

Cross-training is a huge factor in injury prevention because it mitigates the risk of repetitive stress on the body. Remember when we talked about stress fractures? Repeatedly performing the same movements can lead to strain and overuse injuries. For instance, a runner who solely concentrates on running may develop conditions such as shin splints or stress fractures due to the constant impact on their legs. But cross-training helps avoid those by introducing a variety of movements and exercises, allowing overworked muscles and joints to recuperate.

Balancing high-impact and low-impact activities is crucial. While high-impact activities such as running or jumping offer benefits, they can strain the body if overdone. Incorporating low-impact exercises such as swimming, cycling, or yoga provides both recovery and variety. Alternating between high and low-impact exercises allows the body to heal and adapt, reducing the risk of strain or injury. This balance also helps prevent mental burnout and keeps workouts enjoyable and sustainable.

Understanding muscle imbalances is paramount in cross-training. When one muscle group is stronger than its opposing group, it can lead to poor posture and an increased risk of injury. Cross-training, through a variety of exercises, ensures a balanced development of different muscle groups, preventing and addressing these imbalances. Activities like yoga or Pilates promote both strength and flexibility, reducing the risk of muscle imbalances.

Varying the intensity and duration of workouts is another key aspect of cross-training. Constant high-intensity workouts can fatigue the body and increase the risk of injury. Mixing up workout intensity and duration provides the body with the necessary time to recover and adapt, while also maintaining interest and motivation in the fitness routine.

Nutrition for Injury Recovery

When injured, our bodies require additional nutrients to repair and heal due to the increased stress on our system. If we consume the right nutrients, we can accelerate this recovery process.

Protein is a key nutrient for injury recovery because it serves as the building blocks for repairing and building new tissues like your muscles and skin. Foods rich in protein (for example: lean meats, fish, eggs, beans, dairy products, and plant-based sources like nuts) are highly beneficial. The body breaks down these proteins into amino acids, which are then transported to the injured areas to assist in tissue repair and muscle maintenance. Ensuring sufficient protein intake is vital, especially for injuries related to muscles or bones.

Vitamins and minerals also play significant roles in the healing process. Vitamin C, found in fruits and vegetables, is crucial for collagen formation, which aids in tissue repair. Vitamin D, obtainable from sunlight exposure, eggs, and fatty fish, assists in calcium absorption, essential for bone healing. Minerals like calcium, important for both bones and muscle function, and zinc, which facilitates wound healing and tissue building, can be found in dairy products, leafy greens, nuts, whole grains, and seafood. These nutrients contribute to various aspects of the body's recovery.

Carbohydrates are essential for providing the energy needed during the healing process. As energy demands increase while injured, incorporating carbohydrates from whole grains, fruits, and vegetables is crucial. These sources provide healthy carbohydrates that support the recovery process.

Certain foods can reduce inflammation, a common response to injury. Omega-3 fatty acids found in fish like salmon and flaxseeds possess anti-inflammatory properties. Antioxidant-rich foods, such as berries and leafy greens, also aid in combating inflammation and promoting healing.

Lastly, hydration is a critical but often overlooked aspect of injury recovery. We don't often think about it, but water plays a crucial role in facilitating nutrient transportation to the injury site and waste removal. So, it's important to always remember to stay hydrated! Drinking water is essential for an efficient recovery process.

Mind-Body Strategies for Recovery

Imagine you're running in a race. It's a hot day, the sun beating down on you without any clouds to help soften its rays. A breath of wind cools you down as you turn a corner. Your feet fall, heavy, onto the gravel with each step, crunching it. Your legs muscles burn, but you urge them to keep going—the goal is in sight! You push forward. One leg in front of the other, you move closer with each step. Three, two, one—you've finished!

Visualization is more than a simple exercise; it plays a crucial role in injury prevention, management, and recovery. It involves picturing oneself healing, focusing on details like the sensation of strength returning and pain diminishing. This process can boost motivation, reduce anxiety, and foster an optimistic mindset, all vital for a smoother recovery.

Additionally, visualization aids in pain management by triggering the release of endorphins, the body's natural painkillers. This can actually lessen pain perception and make recovery more tolerable. Athletes have long used visualization to enhance performance, and the same principles apply to injury recovery and improving muscle memory and coordination, which accelerates rehabilitation.

Breathwork and relaxation are key components of mind-body recovery strategies, significantly aiding in injury prevention and management, as well as overall well-being. Breathwork involves using controlled breathing to relax your nervous system, which can lower stress, reduce muscle tension, and alleviate injury-related pain. It activates the rest and digest system, diverting energy towards recovery. Deep breathing exercises, like diaphragmatic breathing, can be easily integrated into daily routines.

Relaxation techniques are helpful for counteracting stress-induced impediments to recovery. Progressive muscle relaxation helps release physical tension, particularly beneficial for muscle pain or stiffness. To do it, start by finding a comfortable position, either sitting or lying down in a quiet space. Then, take a few deep breaths to center yourself. Begin at one end of your body, usually the feet, and work your way up. Tense each muscle group for about five seconds and then release it, feeling the tension flow away. Move progressively through each part of the body, paying particular attention to areas that hold stress, like the shoulders and jaw. By gradually working through the body, this practice can help alleviate tension and promote a state of relaxation conducive to recovery.

In addition to progressive muscle relaxation, mindfulness meditation can be a powerful tool in managing stress and fostering a healing environment for the body. To practice mindfulness meditation, find a quiet space and a comfortable position. Close your eyes and bring your attention to your breath. As you inhale and exhale naturally, observe the sensations in your body and the thoughts in your mind without judgment. If your mind wanders, gently bring your focus back to your breath. This practice can be done for as little as five minutes a day and is effective in reducing stress and enhancing overall well-being.

Incorporating these techniques into daily routines, whether during work breaks or before bedtime, can provide long-term benefits in injury recovery.

Finally, biofeedback and neurofeedback introduce innovative recovery strategies focusing on physiological and brain processes. Biofeedback provides real-time data on bodily functions like heart rate and muscle tension, aiding in stress and pain management. Neurofeedback, which focuses on brainwave patterns, has also shown promise in managing chronic pain, migraines, and PTSD. These techniques require professional guidance and offer a non-invasive, side-effect-minimal approach to recovery. They empower individuals to participate actively in their healing process, promoting a holistic approach to injury prevention and management.

Injury Management: PEACE & LOVE

The acronym PEACE & LOVE stands for Protect, Elevate, Avoid, Compress, Educate & Load, Optimization, Vascularization, Exercise. It's a guideline for injury management, particularly for musculoskeletal injuries. It's an updated approach that replaced the older Rest, Ice, Compression, Elevation (RICE) method. This updated acronym emphasizes a more active recovery and recognizes the importance of psychological factors in the healing process.

Let's break down each letter:

- Protect: Avoid activities and movements that cause pain for the first few days after the injury.
- Elevate: Elevate the injured limb higher than the heart as often as possible.
- Avoid Anti-Inflammatory Modalities: Avoid using anti-inflammatory medications and ice as they can delay healing.
- Compress Use compression to reduce swelling.
- Educate: Patients should be educated that recovery is a gradual process.

After the initial PEACE phase, the LOVE approach should be used:

- Load: An injured body part should be loaded gradually and safely.
- Optimism: A positive mindset can influence recovery.
- Vascularization: Cardiovascular activities that are pain-free should be performed to increase blood flow to the injured area.
- Exercise: Exercise should be used to restore mobility, strength, and proprioception, which is the sense that allows you to know where your body parts are in relation to each other and the objects around you.

Other than knowing PEACE & LOVE, it can be incredibly beneficial to take a first aid course. These courses provide essential knowledge and skills that can make a big difference during emergencies and can allow you to minimize the severity of injuries in various situations.

And finally, the importance of seeking professional help for long term injury management and rehabilitation cannot be understated. Healthcare professionals can accurately diagnose your injury, design a tailored rehabilitation program, and closely monitor your progress, ensuring effective and safe recovery. Their expertise, access to the latest rehabilitation techniques, and emotional support can make a significant difference in your journey toward regaining your physical health and overall well-being. This proactive approach minimizes the risk of complications, maximizes your chances of a full recovery, and helps you navigate the physical and psychological challenges that often accompany long-term injuries.

Takeaways

Understanding common injuries equips you with the knowledge to avoid them through proper form, technique, and the integration of cross-training. By familiarizing yourself with the causes and symptoms of various exercise-related ailments, you can take proactive measures to prevent them. Prioritizing correct execution and employing a variety of training methods not only enhances your physical fitness but also acts as a safeguard against the strains and stresses that lead to injury.

This chapter has offered a holistic overview of how to maintain a safe exercise regimen, emphasizing the essentiality of nutrition and hydration, and the benefits of employing mind-body strategies for recovery. 'PEACE & LOVE' provides a modern blueprint for injury management, advocating for an active recovery process supported by a positive psychological outlook. Taking these lessons to heart will not only help you in avoiding and managing injuries but also ensure a quicker, more effective recovery, keeping you on track towards achieving and sustaining a healthy, active lifestyle.

TYPES OF EXERCISES

Strength Training

Strength training, also known as resistance training, is a vital component of a well-rounded fitness regimen. It focuses on muscle growth, power, and resilience. Beyond aesthetics, it offers functional strength that improves daily activities, sports performance, and overall vitality.

Incorporating a variety of exercises, such as as well as compound and isolation exercises, is crucial for a well-rounded routine. Here are some areas that we'll consider:

- Full-Body or Targeted Workouts
- Free Weights or Machines
- Bodyweight and Core Strengthening
- Mobility and Flexibility

Alongside exercise, recognizing the significance of proper nutrition and adequate recovery is essential for optimizing performance, facilitating muscle repair, and supporting growth. Fine-tuning these aspects can accelerate your progress and overall fitness journey.

Choosing the Right Strength Training Exercises

When embarking on a strength training journey, the exercises you select play a pivotal role in shaping your fitness outcomes. Your choices can either propel you toward your goals or hinder your progress. To make informed decisions, it's essential to consider several factors.

One critical decision is the choice between full-body workouts and targeted workouts. Full-body workouts, which involve exercises like squats, deadlifts, and bench presses, engage multiple muscle groups simultaneously. These workouts are highly efficient, offering a comprehensive training session that caters to your entire body's needs. They are particularly advantageous for individuals with limited gym time or beginners aiming to establish a solid foundation of strength.

On the other hand, targeted workouts zero in on specific muscle groups. For example, if your objective is to sculpt your biceps, exercises such as bicep curls and hammer curls would be your go-to options. This approach is tailor-made for individuals with specific aesthetic or strength goals for particular muscle groups. Targeted workouts provide customized routines to address weaknesses or imbalances, making it especially beneficial for athletes involved in sports that demand specialized muscle development, like bodybuilding or powerlifting.

Your choice between these two approaches should align with your unique fitness goals and preferences. Full-body workouts contribute to a well-rounded fitness regimen, while targeted workouts excel at honing in on specific muscle areas.

Another crucial consideration is whether to use free weights or machines. Free weights, like dumbbells and barbells, enhance functional strength and balance by engaging various supporting muscles. In contrast, machines offer stability through their fixed range of motion, making them suitable for beginners or individuals recovering from injuries. Your choice should hinge on your experience level and training objectives, although a combination of both often proves to be the most effective approach.

If you don't have access to free weights or machines, or even if you do and are looking for more variety, then bodyweight exercises could be helpful for your fitness routine. They are indispensable for any well-rounded strength training program. These exercises are versatile and require no equipment, making them accessible to virtually anyone. They improve functional strength and can be tailored to accommodate different fitness levels.

Weights aren't the only aspect of keeping yourself physically fit through exercise. Core strengthening exercises should also hold a prominent place, as they target the muscles in your midsection.

Planks and Russian twists, for instance, not only bolster your spine and posture but also contribute to overall fitness while reducing the risk of injuries.

Additionally, don't overlook the significance of flexibility and mobility exercises like the standing quad stretch or torso twists These exercises are instrumental in maintaining joint health, preventing injuries, and ensuring proper exercise form. Incorporating them into your routine not only enhances muscle function but also promotes fluid joint movement, which is essential for optimizing your strength training efforts.

Lastly, grasp the importance of two key principles: progression and variation. Gradually increasing exercise intensity is fundamental to muscle growth, while constantly changing your routine prevents your body from adapting and keeps your workouts engaging. Both these principles are essential for sustained strength development and warding off workout monotony.

Muscle Mass vs. Strength

In strength training, it's essential to grasp the distinction between muscle mass and strength to set appropriate training goals and methods. Muscle mass is all about size and volume, often seen in bodybuilders with well-defined muscles. Building muscle mass involves a combination of resistance training, sufficient protein intake, and calorie consumption, resulting in larger muscles and a more "buff" appearance.

Strength, on the other hand, focuses on the muscles' ability to exert force, regardless of their size. It's typically measured by the amount of weight one can lift in exercises like bench pressing or squatting. Strength is derived from muscle contraction efficiency and can improve through neurological adaptations and better technique, without necessarily leading to increased muscle size.

Muscle hypertrophy, which involves increasing muscle size, plays a central role in building muscle mass. This process is initiated through resistance training or weightlifting, which creates microtears in muscle fibers. As these fibers heal, they become thicker and stronger. Adequate protein intake is a vital component of this process. For muscle hypertrophy, a common approach is to perform higher repetitions (typically eight to twelve) with moderate to heavy weights.

In contrast, strength development relies on neuromuscular adaptations, which entail changes in the nervous system and muscle communication. These adaptations enhance muscle coordination and motor unit recruitment (which measures active muscle fibers), improving strength without significant muscle size increase. Key factors include more efficient motor unit recruitment and coordinated muscle contractions, often occurring before visible muscle growth is noticeable.

For muscle mass-oriented training, programs like the bodybuilding split routine and high-volume training are designed to stimulate muscle growth. These programs incorporate progressive overload, compound exercises, and a protein-rich diet to maximize muscle hypertrophy.

On the other hand, strength-focused training programs such as the "5x5 program" and powerlifting training prioritize lifting heavy weights with lower repetitions to build strength. Strongman training introduces functional strength elements, and periodization plays a crucial role in these programs, dividing training into different phases with varying focuses. But remember! To achieve significant strength gains, you must also have adequate rest and recovery.

The realm of strength training is vast and varied, offering a multitude of pathways depending on your individual goals and preferences. We've explored the essential components, from understanding the difference between muscle mass and strength to choosing the right mix of exercises.

The key to a successful strength training program lies in balancing variety with consistency, as well as understanding the importance of both muscle development and functional strength. Whether you aim for muscle hypertrophy with high-rep routines or strength enhancement through low-reps and heavy weightlifting, incorporating a blend of full-body, targeted, compound, and isolation exercises will lead to well-rounded fitness.

Cardiovascular Conditioning

Cardiovascular health is an essential aspect of your overall well-being, and understanding the nuances of cardiovascular conditioning can be a game-changer. In this chapter, we delve into two pivotal forms of cardiovascular exercise: Zone 2 Cardiovascular Exercises and VO2 Max Training. Zone 2 training focuses on moderate-intensity exercise in which it optimizes heart efficiency and enhances endurance through a balanced approach. VO2 Max Training, on the other hand, pushes the body to its aerobic limits, significantly boosting endurance and cardiovascular capacity. Both methods offer unique benefits and challenges, and comprehending their roles in fitness can lead to improved health and performance.

Zone 2 Cardiovascular Exercises

Zone 2 cardiovascular conditioning, often referred to as Zone 2 training, is a moderate-intensity exercise method aimed at improving heart and lung efficiency. This training occurs at an intensity where one can maintain a conversation, typically between 60% and 70% of your maximum heart rate. It's a balanced effort that enhances cardiovascular health by making the heart more efficient at pumping blood, delivering oxygen, and removing waste from muscles, thus reducing the risk of heart diseases such as hypertension and coronary artery disease.

A key benefit of Zone 2 cardio is its role in fat metabolism. Exercising at this intensity primarily uses fat as the energy source, aiding in weight loss and body composition improvement. This training also builds endurance, enabling athletes and those in endurance sports to sustain effort over extended periods and improve performance.

Unlike high-intensity workouts, Zone 2 cardiovascular conditioning is less likely to cause overtraining or injury, offering a safe and sustainable way to enhance fitness for people of various ages and fitness levels. It's a holistic approach to fitness, focusing on heart health, fat burning, endurance enhancement, and injury risk reduction.

Heart rate monitoring is vital in Zone 2 exercises because it helps you maintain the correct workout intensity. Methods range from checking your pulse manually to using fitness trackers or smart-watches. These devices provide real-time data and can alert users when they deviate from the Zone 2 range. Monitoring ensures that your exercising remains within the 60-70% maximum heart rate range, both avoiding overtraining and maximizing the benefits of Zone 2 training.

Gradually increasing workout duration and intensity while listening to the body's response is crucial for a positive and effective training experience. For beginners, starting Zone 2 workouts involves calculating the maximum heart rate by subtracting age from 220 and then working within 60-70% of this rate. Starting with low-impact activities like walking or cycling for 20-30 minutes, three to four times a week is recommended.

If regular Zone 2 workouts aren't pushing your limits, then you can move on to advanced Zone 2 training. This method is for those with a solid cardiovascular base who seek to enhance their performance. It involves longer workouts, sometimes exceeding 90 minutes, and may include interval training with short bursts of higher intensity. For example, you could incorporate hill workouts into a longer training routine. Advanced practitioners often use sophisticated heart rate monitoring and vary their training to challenge the cardiovascular system further. This level of training requires dedication, discipline, and possibly professional guidance to optimize your performance and achieve specific fitness goals.

VO2 Max Training

VO2 max training, also known as maximal oxygen consumption training, is essential for cardiovascular conditioning. It aims to improve your body's ability to use oxygen efficiently during physical activity, thereby enhancing endurance and stamina. This type of training pushes your cardiovascular system to its limits by elevating your heart rate to near its maximum capacity for extended periods of time. As a result, your body transports and utilizes oxygen better, allowing your heart, lungs, and muscles to work more effectively together.

The benefits of VO2 max training are substantial. It not only improves cardiovascular fitness but also reduces the risk of heart-related diseases, such as hypertension and coronary artery disease. By enhancing endurance and stamina, it benefits various physical activities like running, cycling, and team sports. Moreover, this training positively impacts daily life by making routine tasks feel less taxing. Additionally, VO2 max training is effective in weight management and fat loss due to increased calorie burn during and after high-intensity workouts.

Measuring your maximum oxygen intake (VO2 max) is crucial for understanding and tracking your cardiovascular fitness progress. More specifically, you need to track the maximum amount of oxygen your body can use during intense exercise, as it is a key indicator of aerobic capacity and endurance. But how do you find this measurement? There are multiple ways to find your VO2 max, such as prediction equations based on personal data, wearable fitness trackers, or a graded test in a lab. Though varying in precision, these methods help provide data that lets you set realistic fitness goals and monitor your progress.

Several factors influence VO2 max, including genetics, age, sex, fitness level, and environmental conditions like altitude and temperature. For example, genetics plays a significant role, but improvements are possible through training regardless of genetic predisposition. As you get older, generally your VO2 max declines, but regular exercise can slow this process. Men typically have a higher VO2 max than women, which is attributed to muscle mass and hormonal differences. Those with a history of consistent aerobic exercise usually have higher VO2 max levels. Lastly, exercising in environments like high altitudes or extreme temperatures can temporarily affect VO2 max.

One of the best ways to improve your VO2 max is through exercise. There are several options, so keep in mind your fitness level, goals, and preferences. In terms of training strategies, there are various methods to improve VO2 max and cardiovascular conditioning:

- High-Intensity Interval Training (HIIT): This is a popular method involving short, intense exercise bursts alternated with rest periods. Tabata, a form of HIIT, consists of 20 seconds of maximum effort followed by 10 seconds of rest, repeated for four minutes.
- Reduced-Exertion High-Intensity Training (REHIT): REHIT focuses on very brief, intense sprints with longer rest periods. This makes it a time-efficient option for improving VO2 max.
- Fartlek Training: This technique offers a more flexible approach, combining varying intensities within a single workout.
- Other Methods: There are many other exercises that can contribute to developing your VO2 max, such as continuous endurance training, tempo runs, and circuit training.

In summary, VO2 max training is a key component of cardiovascular fitness that focuses on enhancing your body's use of oxygen during exercise. It offers numerous benefits, such as improved heart health, endurance, and weight management. Measuring VO2 max helps in setting fitness goals and monitoring progress, while understanding its influencing factors can allow for a more tailored training approach. With various training strategies available, individuals can select the method that best suits their needs and preferences.

Zone 2 Cardiovascular Exercises and VO2 Max Training are integral components of a comprehensive fitness regimen. Zone 2 training, with its emphasis on moderate intensity and endurance, caters to a wide range of fitness levels, promoting heart health and efficient fat metabolism. VO2 Max Training, characterized by high-intensity workouts, elevates one's aerobic capacity and stamina, contributing significantly to cardiovascular fitness.

So, what are you waiting for? By incorporating these methods into your routine, you can achieve a balanced approach to cardiovascular health, enhancing not only your physical performance but also your overall quality of life. Understanding and applying these concepts paves the way for a healthier, more active lifestyle.

Flexibility and Balance

Flexibility and balance are key aspects of maintaining a healthy, active lifestyle, especially as we age. Our bodies undergo numerous changes, and staying limber and balanced can greatly impact our overall well-being and day-to-day life. This chapter delves into the various methods and exercises that enhance flexibility and balance, ranging from static and dynamic stretching to balance-focused exercises and the holistic practice of yoga. Understanding these techniques and incorporating them into your routines can lead to improved mobility, reduced risk of falls and injuries, and a heightened sense of mental clarity and relaxation.

Dynamic vs. Static Stretching

Static stretching involves holding a specific position for a set time to stretch your muscles. It's effective for improving flexibility, as holding a stretch allows muscles to relax and lengthen over time. As the muscles relax, they release tension, which is beneficial after intense workouts or prolonged sitting. Stretching relaxed muscles can also lead to an also enhanced range of motion, making joint movements more comfortable. It's also excellent for relaxation in general! Take deep breaths while stretching, which can help calm your mind and reduce stress.

Dynamic stretching differs significantly from static stretching. It involves moving your body through a range of motions, serving as an active way to prepare your muscles for physical activity. This type of stretching increases blood flow and heart rate, delivering more oxygen and nutrients to your muscles. Because dynamic stretching focuses on stretching and contrasting muscles simultaneously, it can also improve flexibility, though in a different manner than static stretching. The movement of dynamic stretching enhances your range of motion and mobility, which is vital for sports requiring agility. This type of stretching even has the added benefit of improving your coordination and balance because its movement activates your nervous system.

When warming up for physical activities, choosing between dynamic and static stretching is crucial. Dynamic stretching is akin to a warm-up dance, as it gradually increases your joint motion range through active movements like leg swings or lunges. This does a great job of increasing your heart rate and blood flow, preparing your muscles for physical demands, and enhancing your coordination. It makes sense, then, that dynamic stretching is particularly useful for agility-based activities.

On the other hand, for a cool down, you might turn to static stretching, i.e. the classic "reach and hold" method. Static stretching helps relax muscles that have become tight and tense, relieving soreness and discomfort. Regular static stretching in your cool-down routine can increase long-term flexibility, crucial for joint health and injury prevention. Additionally, static stretching offers mental relaxation benefits by aiding in stress reduction and creating a sense of calm post-workout. It's important to perform static stretching when muscles are warm so that you maximize benefits while minimizing injury risks. So, while it does improve long-term flexibility, static stretching might temporarily decrease muscle strength and power, making it less ideal for a pre-activity warm-up and the perfect choice for a cool down.

Balance Exercises

Balance exercises play a crucial role in maintaining an active and healthy lifestyle by improving your stability, coordination, and overall balance. From simple to complex, these exercises cater to various fitness levels and preferences:

- Single-Leg Balance: Stand on one foot, lifting the other slightly off the ground, and try to maintain balance as long as possible. This strengthens leg and core muscles and enhances proprioception, your body's spatial awareness.
- Tandem Walk: Walk heel to toe in a straight line, akin to walking on a tightrope. It boosts balance, coordination, and ankle strength, aiding in everyday activities.
- Bosu Ball or Balance Board: These exercises involve standing on an unstable surface, demanding more muscle work to maintain steadiness. This improves balance and stability over time.
- Yoga and Tai Chi: These both include various balance exercises. Yoga poses like the tree or warrior III involve balancing on one leg in different positions, while tai chi's slow, flowing movements enhance balance, coordination, and flexibility. Both practices promote physical balance and mental relaxation.
- Dynamic Balance Exercises: These involve incorporating movement while still maintaining your balance. Activities like leg swings, heel-to-toe walks, and hopping on one foot challenge your balance in real-life, on-the-move scenarios.

When starting balance exercises, it's essential to match your current fitness level and progress to more challenging exercises gradually to avoid injury.

To enhance balance workouts, various equipment can be utilized.

- Bosu Ball: This is a half-exercise ball attached to a platform, which allows for diverse exercises like squats or lunges on the flat side and one-foot balancing on the rounded side.

- Balance Board: This resembles a wheel-less skateboard, strengthens leg muscles and improves proprioception.
- Stability Ball: A device used for core-engaging exercises.
- Balance Discs: Small discs that provide instability underfoot, strengthening lower leg muscles and aiding ankle injury prevention.
- Resistance Bands: Rubberlike bands that add resistance to balance exercises, engaging more muscle groups.
- Yoga Props: Objects like blocks and straps assist in achieving balance in various poses.

As with other types of exercise, it's important to be adaptable. Progressive overload is a fundamental fitness principle applicable to balance training. It involves gradually making exercises more challenging to continue improving. This can be done by increasing exercise duration, altering intensity, adding or removing equipment, or adjusting repetitions and sets. However, this should be done sensibly to avoid injury.

Balance can also be improved through daily activities. Look for ways to incorporate balance into your daily routine. During an everyday task like brushing your teeth, you could balance on one foot. Or maybe while you walk your dog, you could practice walking heel to toe. Stand up from your computer without using the hand supports, balance while in line at checkout, and use stairs whenever possible. Once you start looking, there are all kinds of ways to integrate exercise into your daily routine. But always remember to exercise caution and use support if needed, especially for those new to balance exercises or with balance issues.

Yoga

Yoga is celebrated for its remarkable ability to enhance balance and flexibility, attracting many to explore why it's so effective. The secret lies in yoga's unique blend of movement and mindfulness. Each yoga session involves various poses that require reaching, twisting, and bending, gently stretching and lengthening muscles as you do so. This consistent practice increases joint and muscle flexibility, making the body more supple and reducing injury risks in daily life.

Yoga also bolsters balance by strengthening core muscles in the abdomen and lower back. As you maintain steady yoga poses, these core muscles are engaged, enhancing your stability and balance in everyday activities. The practice also fosters mindfulness because it heightens awareness of body alignment and balance.

Healthy, mobile joints are essential for free movement and balance. The controlled movements of yoga lubricate joints, aiding mobility and preventing stiffness. If you struggle with arthritis, this aspect would be particularly beneficial!

Mental clarity and relaxation, indirect benefits of yoga, also contribute to improved balance and flexibility. Mental stress and tension can lead to physical stiffness and imbalance. Yoga's deep breathing and mindfulness techniques help reduce stress, allowing the body to move more freely.

Yoga extends its benefits beyond balance and flexibility. It's a key tool in stress reduction, teaching relaxation through deep breathing and mindfulness. This lowers stress hormone levels, fostering calmness. Regular practice improves posture, awareness of spinal alignment, and overall physical bearing. Furthermore, yoga enhances strength and endurance by working various muscle groups and building muscular strength, which improves your overall physical performance and reduces your risk of becoming injured.

Yoga's mental benefits include improved concentration and focus, as it trains the mind to stay present. This can enhance concentration in work or study. It also promotes better sleep, which means it's particularly helpful for people with insomnia or sleep difficulties. Even better, yoga fosters a sense of community and belonging through yoga classes or groups, boosting mental and emotional well-being.

Yoga's diversity is apparent through its various types that each offer unique benefits:

- Hatha Yoga: This style is ideal for beginners, focuses on basic poses and breathing, improving flexibility and promoting relaxation.
- Vinyasa Yoga: If you're looking for something more dynamic, this style offers a more flowing sequence that builds strength, endurance, and flexibility.
- Kundalini Yoga: This exercise aims for spiritual awakening by combining dynamic postures, breathing techniques, and meditation.
- Restorative Yoga: These stretches are good for stress relief and calming yourself. It uses props for passive poses, ideal for anxiety or insomnia sufferers.
- Bikram or Hot Yoga: Perform this yoga in a heated room, as it focuses on detoxification and flexibility enhancement through a structured sequence of poses.
- Ashtanga Yoga: This is the most physically demanding style, which focuses on strength, flexibility, and stamina, suitable for those who enjoy a disciplined and challenging practice.

In summary, yoga's myriad benefits for improving balance, flexibility, stress reduction, posture, strength, mental focus, sleep, and community, along with its variety of styles, make it a comprehensive practice for enhancing physical and mental well-being.

The importance of flexibility and balance in our daily lives cannot be overstated. Through a combination of static and dynamic stretching, balance exercises, and the holistic practice of yoga, individuals can achieve improved physical stability, mental clarity, and an overall sense of well-being. Whether it's through simple daily activities or structured exercise routines, incorporating these elements into our lives can lead to significant long-term health benefits. As we age, these practices become even more crucial, helping to maintain mobility, prevent injuries, and ensure a higher quality of life.

Active Recovery Techniques

Active recovery involves engaging in low-intensity exercises or activities after intense workouts or injuries. It promotes blood circulation, reduces muscle soreness, and helps maintain flexibility. All of these aid in quicker recovery while preventing stiffness and enhancing overall fitness.

We have already covered a couple of ways to engage in active recovery in other parts of this guide. Dynamic stretching is one method, along with various forms of light exercise, such as walking or low-intensity swimming.

The rest of this section will explore additional methods to expedite your recovery in order to ensure that you are in top condition for your next training day.

Self-Myofascial Release

Self-myofascial release (SMR) is a technique where you apply pressure to your muscles and fascia (important connective tissues) to alleviate tightness and enhance flexibility. It's like a self-administered deep tissue massage, often done with tools or body weight. This method is beneficial for relieving muscle soreness and tightness, which commonly occur after physical activity. SMR helps to loosen up knots in the muscles, promoting blood flow and improving flexibility.

Additionally, SMR can improve your range of motion. Tight muscles and fascia can limit movement, but regular SMR practice helps break down adhesions in your fascia, allowing you to stretch and move more easily. This is particularly advantageous for athletes and those seeking to boost their overall mobility. Moreover, SMR can reduce the risk of injury! Tightness can often lead to strains during physical activities, and SMR reduces that likelihood by maintaining muscle balance and loosening your tight muscles and fascia.

So, how do you perform SMR? There are various tools and techniques that you'll need. A foam roller is effective for large muscle groups like the quadriceps and hamstrings. You roll over the muscle with the foam roller to knead out tight spots. For smaller or harder-to-reach muscles, a lacrosse ball or tennis ball can target specific trigger points, like under the shoulder blade or in the calves. For deeper muscle groups like the glutes or hips, a massage stick is beneficial, and specialized tools like spiky massage balls can offer deeper relief in various body parts.

To make the most of SMR, you'll need to do more than massage the area. Breathing techniques can enhance SMR's effectiveness. Deep diaphragmatic breathing helps relax muscles, while synchronized breathing aligns your breath with the movement, aiding in control and consistency. Mindful breathing—remember that this means focusing on slow, deliberate breaths—helps you connect with your body and adjust the pressure as needed.

It's important to differentiate between pain and discomfort in SMR. Discomfort is normal, indicating tension release, while pain suggests something is wrong, and you should reassess your technique.

Starting lightly and gradually increasing pressure ensures you won't hurt yourself on accident. Listening to your body is key! Stop or adjust if pain occurs. The duration of SMR sessions varies, but starting with one to two minutes per muscle group and potentially increasing to five to ten minutes can be effective. Frequency depends on individual needs and can range from several times a week to daily, either as a warm-up or cool-down activity.

Common mistakes in SMR include using too much pressure, rolling too quickly, improper form, neglecting proper breathing, and not staying hydrated. Avoiding these mistakes ensures a more effective and safe SMR practice. Remember, SMR is a tool for recovery and maintenance and should be part of a balanced training regimen.

Professional Massage

Active recovery techniques are essential in recovering from strenuous physical activities, and professional massages stand out as one of the most effective methods. Different types of massages cater to various needs, and selecting the right one is crucial for effective recovery. Below are some options you could choose from:

- Swedish Massage: This type of massage is excellent for active recovery. It uses gentle strokes, kneading, and light tapping to relax the body, reduce muscle tension, and improve circulation. This type of massage is ideal after a tough workout or sports event.
- Sports Massage: This massage is tailored for athletes. It focuses on muscles stressed during physical activities, using deep tissue techniques to alleviate soreness, reduce inflammation, and enhance flexibility. This is especially beneficial for those engaged in regular, rigorous training or sports activities.
- Deep Tissue Massage: For individuals with specific muscle pain or discomfort, deep tissue massage is advisable. This technique uses more pressure to reach deeper muscle layers and connective tissue, helping to release chronic tension, break down scar tissue, and improve mobility. It's particularly useful for chronic pain or injury recovery.
- Trigger Point Therapy: This is a more precise massage that can also play a significant role in active recovery. It targets tight knots in the muscles that cause pain and restrict movement. Applying pressure to these trigger points helps muscles relax and speeds up recovery.

Choosing the right massage depends on your individual needs and active recovery goals. Whether it's for relaxation, addressing specific muscle issues, targeting deep muscle tension, or releasing tight knots, the right massage technique can significantly aid in recovery.

Don't forget to think about the timing of your massage! Generally, it's best to schedule a massage a day or two after strenuous exercise, allowing your body to recover naturally from the immediate workout stress. Timing your massage too soon or too late could either cause discomfort or diminish its effectiveness. Personal preferences and schedule should also be considered, as well as your long-term training goals. Regular massages can be incorporated into your routine for ongoing muscle maintenance and injury prevention.

Lastly, choosing a qualified massage therapist is crucial. Look for a licensed and certified therapist, consider their experience and expertise, communicate openly about your needs and expectations, seek referrals and reviews, and trust your instincts. A skilled therapist will ensure a positive and effective massage experience, tailored to your recovery needs.

Cold Therapy

Cold therapy, including ice baths, cryotherapy chamber sessions, and cold pack applications, is an effective method for active recovery. These techniques help in reducing muscle soreness, inflammation, and speeding up recovery after intense physical activities or injuries.

To take an effective ice bath, start by filling a bathtub or a large container with cold water, ideally at a temperature of 50-60 °F (10-15 °C). Before entering the bath, warm up your body with light exercises or stretches for about five to ten minutes. Then, gradually add ice to the water, using ice cubes or ice packs, to a comfortable temperature. Slowly lower yourself into the ice bath, starting with your feet, and aim to stay immersed for about ten to fifteen minutes, moving your limbs gently to encourage circulation. Afterward, exit the bath and warm up with a towel or blanket. It's important to listen to your body and avoid prolonged exposure.

Cryotherapy chamber sessions offer another form of cold therapy. In these sessions, you step into a chamber with temperatures as low as -200 °F (-129 °C) for two to four minutes. You'll wear minimal clothing along with protective gear like gloves and socks. During the session, keep moving to maintain blood flow. Afterward, warm up slowly. These sessions are known for reducing inflammation and muscle soreness and providing a rejuvenating effect.

For managing injuries, cold therapy can be applied through ice packs or cold-water immersion. When using ice packs, place a barrier like a cloth between the pack and your skin, and apply it for about fifteen to twenty minutes every two to three hours during the first forty eight hours post-injury. Cold water immersion is useful for larger injuries like sprains, where soaking the affected area in cold water can help reduce swelling. Combining cold therapy with compression can also be effective. It's crucial to consult a healthcare professional for proper guidance and to avoid prolonged exposure to extreme cold, which can cause tissue damage.

Overall, cold therapy is a valuable tool in active recovery, whether it's for general muscle recovery or injury management.

Heat Therapy

On the other end of the temperature spectrum, sauna sessions, hot baths, heat packs, heating pads, and contrast therapy are also all effective heat therapy techniques for active recovery. Each method offers unique benefits and requires specific practices for optimal results.

Sauna sessions involve sitting in a heated room, typically between 160°F to 200°F. This induces sweating, helping to remove toxins and metabolic waste through the skin. It also increases blood circulation, which aids muscle recovery and reduces soreness. Beginners should start with 10-15 minute sessions and gradually increase the duration. Don't forget to drink water! Hydration is vital before and after a session to replace lost fluids. Comfortable clothing is recommended, and it's important to listen to your body and leave the sauna if you begin feeling lightheaded or uncomfortable.

Hot baths, with temperatures ranging from 100 °F to 104 °F, are another form of heat therapy. Soaking in warm water relaxes your muscles and releases tension, which is beneficial after intense workouts. A 15-30 minute soak is ideal, though again, it's important to remember to drink water and hydrate during this activity. If you want, adding Epsom salt or essential oils can enhance the therapeutic effects. After the bath, you'll want to gradually cool down to avoid shocking your body.

Heat packs and heating pads provide targeted warmth that is particularly effective for localized muscle pain or tension. A safe temperature range is 104 °F to 113 °F. It's important to start with a lower setting and gradually increase to a temperature that you're comfortable with. Always place a fabric layer between your skin and the heating device, and limit application to 15-20 minutes. Avoid heat therapy immediately after physical activity and ensure you're using the device safely by following manufacturer guidelines and checking the product for any damage before you use it.

Contrast therapy combines heat and cold treatments. First you begin with a heat source like a warm towel or heating pad for about 15-20 minutes to relax muscles and increase blood flow. Then you follow up with a cold source like an ice pack for 10-15 minutes to reduce inflammation and numb pain. Alternate between heat and cold for two to three rounds, finishing with cold therapy. This method stimulates circulation and speeds up recovery, but always listen to your body's response and consult a healthcare professional if you have any medical conditions.

These various heat therapy techniques, when practiced correctly, can significantly aid in active recovery. They help with muscle relaxation, improving circulation, reducing soreness, and promoting overall muscle recovery. The key is to always adhere to the best practices such as appropriate duration, temperature control, hydration, and listening to your body's signals. These methods are beneficial but should be used cautiously, especially by those new to heat therapy or with specific health conditions. Remember, the goal of these therapies is to aid recovery in a comfortable and safe manner, enhancing your overall physical well-being.

Takeaways

When it comes to strength training, incorporating a mix of full-body and targeted workouts, free weights, machines, and bodyweight exercises can lead to a comprehensive regimen that enhances muscle growth, functional strength, and overall vitality.

Tailoring exercise selection to personal fitness goals—whether to enhance overall strength or to concentrate on specific muscle groups—is fundamental for meaningful progress. The synergy between nutrition and adequate recovery underscores the need for a well-rounded regimen that fuels performance and facilitates muscle repair, thereby accelerating fitness journeys.

A clear distinction between muscle mass and strength guides the focus of training, with muscle hypertrophy contributing to size and volume, and neuromuscular adaptations enhancing the ability to exert force. Cardiovascular conditioning, through Zone 2 and VO2 Max training, is pivotal for endurance and heart efficiency, offering a spectrum of benefits that cater to various fitness levels and goals. Flexibility and balance are also crucial, with dynamic and static stretching, alongside targeted balance exercises, maintaining healthy movement, preventing injuries, and enhancing stability, with practices like yoga and Tai Chi providing effective pathways to these ends.

Active recovery techniques, including dynamic stretching, self-myofascial release, and the application of cold and heat, are essential for sustaining training momentum and facilitating muscle recuperation. These practices prepare the body for ongoing physical demands. Ultimately, this comprehensive perspective on fitness underscores the importance of addressing the multiple facets of physical health—strength, endurance, flexibility, balance, and recovery—to not only cultivate physical prowess but also to enrich overall life quality.

PERSONALIZING YOUR FITNESS JOURNEY

Now that you have a solid foundation of knowledge, it's time to put it into practice. In this section, we will guide you through the practical steps of crafting your own fitness journey.

Considerations

Before you start creating your personal fitness plan, there are several factors you need to consider. We have discussed most of these, but here's a checklist of six considerations for you to think about as you begin to brainstorm for your own plan:

- Consider Your Interests: It's crucial for motivation that your fitness plan aligns with activities you genuinely enjoy. Whether it's running, swimming, dancing, or playing a sport, choosing activities you find interesting makes it more likely you'll stay committed to your plan over the long term.
- Define Your Goals: Clearly outlining your fitness objectives, whether it's weight loss, muscle gain, improved endurance, or overall health, provides motivation and helps tailor your plan to achieve those desired outcomes.
- Account for Your Personal Abilities: Assess your current fitness level, skillset, age, and any pre-existing injuries or health conditions. This ensures that your plan is safe, realistic, and suited to your individual needs.
- Consider the Equipment or Facilities: Whether it's free weights, a gym membership, or a running trail, having the right resources is crucial for the success of your fitness plan.
- Decide About a Social Aspect: Having a network of friends, family, or workout partners can provide motivation, encouragement, and accountability. Conversely, if you prefer to train alone, this preference will greatly influence the activities you choose.

- Evaluate Your Schedule: Determine how much time you can realistically dedicate to exercise each week. Balancing work, family, and other commitments with your fitness routine is essential for maintaining consistency.

Specialized Workouts

There are literally hundreds, if not thousands, of different ways to exercise. In this discussion, we'll touch on a few popular methods to provide some ideas for what you might incorporate into your personal fitness routine.

Crossfit

CrossFit is a fitness program that's gained popularity for its intense and varied workouts. It's not just about lifting weights or running on a treadmill. Instead, CrossFit combines different types of exercises to give you a well-rounded workout. You might find yourself doing things like lifting weights, jumping rope, or doing push-ups and sit-ups. The idea is to work different muscle groups and improve overall fitness.

One of the key elements of CrossFit is weightlifting. This involves using barbells, dumbbells, or kettlebells to lift weights in various ways. You might do exercises like deadlifts, squats, or overhead presses. Weightlifting helps to build strength and muscle mass, which can improve your overall fitness and make everyday activities easier.

Aerobic exercises are also an important part of CrossFit. These are activities that get your heart pumping and your blood flowing. You might do things like running, rowing, or jumping jacks. Aerobic exercises help to improve your cardiovascular health, increase your endurance, and burn calories.

Functional movements are another key component of CrossFit. These are exercises that mimic movements you might do in everyday life, like squatting down to pick something up or lifting a heavy object overhead. Functional movements help to improve your flexibility, balance, and coordination, making you better able to perform daily tasks and reducing your risk of injury.

What sets CrossFit apart from other workout programs is its focus on intensity. CrossFit workouts are designed to be challenging and push you to your limits. You might do a series of exercises in a short amount of time, or try to complete as many repetitions as possible in a set period. This intensity helps to maximize your results and keep your workouts interesting and engaging.

Overall, CrossFit is a popular and effective workout program that combines weightlifting, aerobic exercises, and functional movements to improve strength, endurance, and flexibility. By incorporating a variety of exercises and focusing on intensity, CrossFit offers a comprehensive approach to fitness that can help you reach your goals and improve your overall health and well-being.

High-Intensity Interval Training

High-Intensity Interval Training, commonly known as HIIT, is a workout method designed to be both time-efficient and effective. It involves alternating between short bursts of intense exercise and brief rest periods. This means you work hard for a short amount of time, then take a quick break before repeating the cycle.

One of the great things about HIIT is its adaptability. You can customize HIIT workouts to fit your fitness level and preferences. Whether you prefer running, cycling, bodyweight exercises, or using equipment like kettlebells or dumbbells, there's a HIIT workout for you. This versatility makes HIIT accessible to a wide range of people, from beginners to advanced athletes.

HIIT workouts are known for their ability to help individuals burn calories quickly. The high-intensity intervals push your body to work harder, which can lead to a greater calorie burn compared to steady-state cardio exercises like jogging or cycling at a moderate pace. Additionally, HIIT has been shown to increase your metabolism, which means you continue to burn calories even after you've finished your workout.

Another benefit of HIIT is its positive impact on cardiovascular health. By pushing your heart rate up during the intense intervals, HIIT workouts help to improve your cardiovascular fitness and strengthen your heart. Over time, this can lead to better endurance and a reduced risk of heart disease.

P90X

P90X is a structured fitness program that's all about challenging yourself with a variety of exercises. It's designed for people who want a comprehensive workout regimen that targets different aspects of fitness. In P90X, you'll find a mix of exercises including strength training, cardio, yoga, and plyometrics.

One of the key features of P90X is its emphasis on muscle strength and endurance. Through resistance training exercises like lifting weights or using resistance bands, P90X helps to build and tone muscles, making you stronger and more resilient. This can be especially beneficial for everyday activities and preventing injuries.

Cardiovascular exercise is also an important component of P90X. Activities like jogging, jumping rope, or doing high-intensity interval training help to improve your heart health and increase your endurance. By incorporating cardio into your workout routine, P90X helps you burn calories and improve your overall fitness level.

Yoga is another element of P90X that sets it apart from other fitness programs. Yoga helps to improve flexibility, balance, and relaxation, which are important for overall well-being. It also provides a mental break from the intensity of the other exercises, helping you to de-stress and focus on your breath and body.

Plyometrics, or jump training, is a challenging aspect of P90X that focuses on explosive movements to build power and agility. Exercises like jumping squats, burpees, and box jumps help to improve your athletic performance and coordination, while also burning calories and increasing your heart rate.

P90X is a structured fitness program designed to provide a challenging and comprehensive workout regimen. By incorporating a variety of exercises including strength training, cardio, yoga, and plyometrics, P90X helps to enhance muscle strength, endurance, flexibility, and overall fitness. Whether you're a beginner or an experienced athlete, P90X offers a customizable and effective way to achieve your fitness goals.

Martial Arts

Martial arts, like karate and jiu-jitsu, provide more than just self-defense skills—they offer a complete workout for the entire body. These disciplines emphasize not only combat techniques but also physical fitness, agility, balance, and mental discipline through a variety of martial techniques and forms.

One of the primary benefits of practicing martial arts is the improvement in physical fitness. Techniques such as punches, kicks, blocks, and grappling movements engage various muscle groups, promoting strength, endurance, and flexibility. Through repetitive practice, practitioners develop greater control over their bodies, enhancing their overall physical capabilities.

Agility and balance are also key components of martial arts training. Practitioners learn to move swiftly and efficiently, reacting to opponents' movements with speed and precision. This agility and balance training not only improves martial arts performance but also carries over into everyday activities, reducing the risk of falls and injuries.

Moreover, martial arts training fosters mental discipline and focus. Practitioners must remain attentive and disciplined during training sessions, following instructions carefully and executing techniques with precision. This mental aspect of martial arts helps individuals develop concentration, resilience, and self-control, which can be applied beyond the dojo to various aspects of life.

By incorporating self-defense skills, full-body workouts, and mental discipline, disciplines like karate and jiu-jitsu provide practitioners with the tools to improve their overall health and quality of life. Whether for self-defense, fitness, or personal growth, martial arts offer a rewarding and fulfilling journey for individuals of all ages and fitness levels.

Team Sports

Team sports such as basketball and soccer offer more than just a fun way to stay active—they provide a dynamic platform for improving cardiovascular health, agility, and fostering teamwork. Engaging in these sports not only benefits physical health but also promotes social interaction and enjoyment of exercise.

Participating in team sports involves continuous movement, which contributes to improved cardiovascular health. Running, jumping, and quick changes in direction during gameplay elevate heart rate and enhance endurance over time. Regular participation in team sports can lead to better cardiovascular fitness, reducing the risk of heart disease and improving overall well-being.

Furthermore, team sports require agility and quick reflexes, as players must navigate the field or court, evade opponents, and execute precise movements with speed and coordination. These activities help to develop agility, balance, and coordination, which are essential skills for optimal athletic performance and injury prevention.

Beyond physical benefits, team sports promote teamwork and social interaction. Players learn to communicate effectively, collaborate with teammates, and support each other towards a common goal. These interactions foster a sense of camaraderie and belonging, enhancing social skills and building friendships that extend beyond the playing field.

Moreover, the social aspect of team sports can make exercise more enjoyable and motivating. Being part of a team provides a sense of community and accountability, encouraging regular participation and commitment to physical activity. This social support network can help individuals maintain a consistent exercise routine and derive greater satisfaction from their fitness endeavors.

Engaging in team sports not only improves physical fitness but also enhances social interaction and enjoyment of exercise. Whether playing for recreation or competition, participation in these sports provides numerous benefits for overall health and well-being.

Outdoor Sports

Outdoor sports, like hiking and rock climbing, provide a unique opportunity to connect with nature while enhancing physical fitness. These activities not only challenge muscles and improve endurance but also offer mental relaxation in natural settings.

One of the primary benefits of outdoor sports is the physical challenge they present. Hiking and rock climbing engage various muscle groups throughout the body, including the legs, arms, and core. The uneven terrain and elevation changes encountered during these activities provide a full-body workout, promoting strength, flexibility, and cardiovascular health.

Furthermore, outdoor sports offer a dynamic and immersive experience that can't be replicated in indoor environments. Hiking through scenic trails or scaling rock faces requires concentration, coordination, and problem-solving skills. Negotiating natural obstacles and navigating unfamiliar terrain provide mental stimulation while enhancing physical abilities.

Moreover, outdoor sports provide an opportunity for mental relaxation and stress relief in natural surroundings. Spending time outdoors has been shown to reduce stress levels and improve mood, offering a welcome respite from the pressures of daily life. The tranquility of nature and the sense of awe inspired by natural landscapes can promote mental well-being and rejuvenate the spirit.

Additionally, outdoor sports foster a deeper appreciation for the environment and promote environmental stewardship. As individuals explore natural landscapes and interact with wilderness areas, they develop a greater understanding of the importance of preserving these resources for future generations. This awareness can lead to more sustainable behaviors and a commitment to protecting the natural world.

Outdoor sports combine physical challenge, mental stimulation, and natural relaxation. Engaging in these activities allows you to connect with nature, improve physical fitness, and cultivate a deeper appreciation for the environment. Whether for recreation or adventure, outdoor sports provide numerous benefits for overall health and well-being.

Dance Fitness

Dance fitness programs like Zumba and hip-hop dance offer a lively blend of energetic dance moves and fitness routines. These programs not only provide a fun way to get in shape but also help improve coordination, stamina, and overall fitness levels through rhythmic movements set to music.

One of the key benefits of dance fitness programs is their ability to enhance coordination and agility. Participants are challenged to synchronize their movements with the rhythm of the music, incorporating various steps, twists, and turns. Over time, this practice improves motor skills and spatial awareness, leading to better coordination and fluidity in movement.

Additionally, dance fitness programs contribute to improved stamina and endurance. The continuous movement and cardio-intensive nature of these workouts elevate heart rate and boost cardiovascular fitness. Participants engage in sustained physical activity throughout the session, which helps build stamina and increase endurance over time.

Moreover, dance fitness programs offer a joyful and uplifting atmosphere that makes exercise feel like a celebration rather than a chore. Dancing to lively music and engaging with a supportive community of fellow participants creates a positive and motivating environment. This encourages individuals to stick with their fitness routine and enjoy the process of getting fit.

Furthermore, dance fitness programs provide a creative outlet for self-expression and artistic exploration. Participants have the freedom to express themselves through movement, whether it's through the sultry rhythms of salsa or the high-energy beats of hip-hop. This creative aspect adds an element of enjoyment and fulfillment to the workout experience.

Aquatic Workouts

Aquatic workouts, like water aerobics and swimming, are exercises done in the water. They're great because they're easy on your joints. When you do these workouts, you're moving your body in the water. It's like exercising, but the water supports you, so there's less strain on your joints.

One big benefit of aquatic workouts is they're good for your heart. When you move around in the water, your heart has to work a bit harder to keep you going. This helps make your heart stronger and healthier. Plus, since the water offers resistance, it helps to build up your muscles. You might not even realize it, but just moving your arms and legs in the water is giving them a good workout.

Another cool thing about aquatic workouts is they can help make you more flexible. The water allows you to move your body in ways you might not be able to on land. It's like stretching, but with the added bonus of being in the water. This can be especially helpful if you have stiff joints or if you're recovering from an injury.

Swimming is a popular aquatic workout. It's not only a fun activity but also a great way to exercise your whole body. When you swim, you're using muscles all over, from your arms and legs to your core. Plus, it's a good way to improve your breathing and endurance.

Water aerobics is another fantastic aquatic workout option. It's like doing aerobics, but in the water. You'll do things like jumping jacks, leg lifts, and arm exercises—all while floating in the water. It's a fun and effective way to get your heart pumping and your muscles working.

Overall, aquatic workouts are a fantastic way to stay active and healthy. They're gentle on your joints, good for your heart, and can help improve your flexibility. Whether you're swimming laps or doing water aerobics, you'll get a great workout while having fun in the water. So next time you're looking for a new way to exercise, consider giving aquatic workouts a try!

Yoga

Yoga is a type of exercise that's known for it's mind-body connection, but that's not all its for. When you do yoga, you'll do different poses and breathing exercises that help make your body stronger and more flexible.

One of the main things yoga focuses on is flexibility. When you do yoga poses, you're gently stretching your muscles, which helps make them more flexible over time. This can be really helpful if you're feeling tight or stiff in certain areas of your body.

Balance is another big part of yoga. Many yoga poses require you to balance on one leg or hold yourself in a certain position. This helps improve your balance and coordination, which can be useful in everyday life.

But yoga isn't just about the physical stuff. It's also really good for your mind. When you do yoga, you often focus on your breath and try to quiet your thoughts. This can help reduce stress and make you feel more relaxed and calm.

Overall, yoga is a great way to take care of both your body and your mind. It helps improve flexibility and balance while also promoting relaxation and reducing stress. Whether you're a beginner or an experienced yogi, there are always new poses and techniques to try, making it a versatile and fulfilling practice for people of all ages and fitness levels.

Pilates

Pilates is great for strengthening your core, which is the muscles around your abdomen and back. But it's not just about building a strong core; it's also about improving flexibility and body awareness.

When you do Pilates, you'll do specific movements and exercises that focus on controlling your muscles. These movements are usually slow and controlled, which helps you build strength without straining your body.

One of the great things about Pilates is that it helps improve your posture. By strengthening your core muscles, you can stand up straighter and taller, which can reduce back pain and make you look more confident.

Balance is another important aspect of Pilates. Many Pilates exercises require you to balance on one leg or hold yourself in a certain position, which helps improve your balance and stability.

Overall, Pilates is a fantastic way to strengthen your core, improve your flexibility, and become more aware of your body. Whether you're new to exercise or a seasoned athlete, Pilates offers a variety of exercises that can help you achieve your fitness goals while also promoting better posture and body alignment.

It appears that there was a mix-up with the file; instead of an image, I received a text input. Based on the text provided, it is clear that the discussion revolves around various types of workouts, each with its unique benefits and characteristics. Here's a conclusion and suggestions on how to decide which type of workout might be the best fit:

Choosing the right type of workout depends on your personal fitness goals, preferences, and lifestyle. To decide which workout is best for you, consider the following suggestions:

Identify Your Fitness Goals: If you want to improve cardiovascular health, consider HIIT or team sports. For muscle strength and mass, look at weightlifting aspects of CrossFit or P90X. If flexibility and balance are your targets, yoga or Pilates might be the way to go.

Assess Your Current Fitness Level: Beginners may start with gentler programs like aquatic workouts or yoga to build a fitness base, while more advanced exercisers might prefer the challenge of CrossFit or martial arts.

Consider Your Time Commitment: If you have limited time, HIIT sessions can be more practical. For those who can dedicate more time and want a varied routine, P90X or CrossFit could be suitable.

Think About Enjoyment: It's crucial to enjoy your workout for long-term adherence. If you love being outdoors, consider outdoor sports. If music and dance appeal to you, dance fitness programs could be a perfect fit.

Reflect on Social Preferences: If you thrive in a group setting, team sports, dance fitness, or martial arts provide social interaction. If you prefer solitary activities, individual sports, swimming, or a home workout program like P90X might be better.

Listen to Your Body: Pay attention to any physical limitations or previous injuries. Aquatic workouts or yoga can be excellent low-impact options for those with joint concerns.

By evaluating these factors, you can narrow down your options and choose a workout that aligns with your needs, leading to a more enjoyable and sustainable fitness journey.

Steps to Create Your Training Plan

Throughout this guide, we've delved into the intricacies of crafting a personalized exercise plan tailored to your unique needs and goals. Now, let's recap the key stages to guide you on this fitness journey.

1. Set Clear Fitness Goals: Start by defining your fitness objective, whether you want to focus primarily on weight

loss, muscle gain, improved endurance, or other specific goals.

2. Assess Your Current Fitness Level: Evaluate your current physical condition, including your strength, flexibility, and any limitations or injuries.

3. Determine Your Training Frequency: Decide how many days per week you can commit to exercising, considering your schedule and availability.

4. Select Appropriate Activities: Choose exercises and activities that align with your goals and interests, ensuring you enjoy your workouts.

5. Plan Your Weekly Schedule: Create a weekly workout schedule, allocating specific days for different types of exercises, such as cardio, strength training, and flexibility training.

6. Set Progression Milestones: Define milestones or targets to track your progress over time, such as weight lifted, distance run, or body measurements.

7. Consider Recovery and Rest Days: Include rest days in your plan to allow your body to recover and prevent overtraining.

8. Nutrition and Hydration: Integrate a nutrition and hydration plan that supports your fitness goals, as diet plays a crucial role in your overall success.

9. Adapt and Adjust: Be prepared to adapt your plan as needed, whether it's modifying exercises, increasing intensity, or addressing any setbacks.

10. Seek Professional Guidance: If necessary, consult with a fitness professional, such as a trainer or physiotherapist, for expert advice and guidance in creating your personalized training plan.

Sam Fury's Exercise Routine

In the dynamic world of fitness and personal health, individual routines often vary as much as the goals and preferences of those who adopt them. "Sam Fury's Exercise Routine" offers an insightful peek into a well-structured, adaptable fitness regimen tailored to an individual's unique needs and interests. From martial arts to strength training, and from yoga to swimming, this routine encapsulates a comprehensive approach to fitness, blending various forms of exercise to achieve a balanced and effective workout. With a focus on increasing strength, enhancing endurance, and maintaining overall health, this routine is designed for those who value a well-rounded fitness experience. The regimen is not just about physical workouts; it also incorporates elements like meditation and self-myofascial massage, highlighting the importance of mental well-being and recovery in any fitness journey.

The following is my current training regimen. I have been following this routine for quite some time, though I do make occasional adjustments when I'm injured or traveling. In most cases, this involves replacing pull-ups, swimming, or running with alternative exercises.

To give you some context, here are my six considerations that I used while brainstorming for my own exercise plan:

1. Interests: I enjoy martial arts, running, swimming, strength training, and yoga.
2. Goals: My goals are to increase strength through strength training and improve endurance and speed when running. For everything else, I aim to maintain my current level.
3. Abilities: I consider myself to be in good overall health with an above-average fitness level. I have a decent background in martial arts and am a proficient swimmer.
4. Equipment: For running, all I need is some open space. My strength training requires a pull-up bar and preferably a weighted vest, although I can perform bodyweight exercises

if necessary and simply increase the repetitions. I swim at the beach, and, when I'm traveling, I go for a jog or a ruck instead.

5. Social: I prefer to train alone.
6. Schedule: I typically train first thing in the morning and, while I'm flexible with timing, I aim to keep it under an hour.

My training follows a weekly schedule:

- Day One: VO2 max training
- Day Two: Strength training
- Day Three: Swimming
- Day Four: Strength training
- Day Five: VO2 max
- Day Six: Strength training
- Day Seven: Active rest day

For VO2 max training, I start with a general warm-up that includes dynamic stretching like leg raises. I prefer either interval training with sprints and jogging, or REHIT.

- During interval training, I jog for four minutes and then sprint hard for one minute, repeating this cycle four times.
- For REHIT training, starting from a resting heart rate, I sprint as hard as I can for sixty seconds and then rest for three minutes. I repeat this two to four times depending on the time available. My cool-down consists of yoga and ten minutes of meditation, with the yoga routine and meditations varying from day to day.

My warm-up for strength training involves shadow boxing. Then, I do three to five sets of the following exercises with a weighted vest (the weight remains the same between exercises, except for broad jumps, and I adjust the weight when it becomes too easy):

- Five reps of pull-ups
- Ten reps of dips
- Five reps of full squats
- Twenty reps of push-ups
- Ten reps of single-leg calf raises on each leg
- Five reps of chin-ups
- Ten reps of broad jumps without weight

On my swimming day, I warm up with sun salutations and then swim one kilometer. On my active recovery day, I also do sun salutations, go for a walk (preferably in nature) and do self-myofascial massage. Sometimes I'll go for a professional massage, such as Thai Massage. I also enjoy saunas.

To aid recovery during the training week, I use ice baths.

By combining different forms of exercise such as strength training, running, swimming, and yoga, and aligning them with individual goals and abilities, this routine showcases the effectiveness of a holistic approach to fitness. The inclusion of recovery techniques like ice baths, professional massages, and meditation underscores the importance of rest and mental well-being in achieving fitness goals. This routine, adaptable for those with busy schedules or limited equipment, proves that with dedication and the right approach, maintaining a high level of fitness is achievable for anyone.

CONCLUSION

As you reach the end of this guide, you stand at a pivotal moment in your fitness journey. Armed with the knowledge and strategies from the preceding chapters, you are now prepared to instill a dynamic, adaptable fitness regime into your daily life. This journey, however, is not about reaching a final destination but rather about embracing a continuous process of growth, adjustment, and personal evolution.

Throughout this guide, we have emphasized the importance of adaptability in your fitness routine. The dynamic fitness approach you've learned is more than a set of exercises; it's a mindset that empowers you to stay responsive to your body's needs, your evolving goals, and the inevitable changes life brings. As you move forward, remember that your fitness journey is uniquely yours. It will grow and change as you do, always providing a space for improvement and self-discovery.

As you develop new strengths, make sure to always cultivate balanced exercises. The importance of a well-balanced routine really cannot be overstated. Just as strength and cardiovascular training are vital, so too are flexibility, balance, and active recovery. These elements work in harmony to create a holistic fitness regime that nurtures your body, reduces the risk of injury, and keeps your workouts engaging and effective.

Remember, setbacks and challenges are a natural part of any journey. There may be days when motivation wanes or life's demands seem to overshadow your fitness goals. In these moments, recall the foundational principles of setting realistic goals and maintaining an adaptable mindset. Adjust your routine as needed, but always keep your overarching vision in sight.

You've already come so far! take a moment to reflect on your achievements: You have taken crucial steps towards a healthier, more balanced lifestyle. Continue to draw upon the lessons and strategies you've learned and remain open to new ideas and approaches that resonate with your evolving fitness journey.

Finally, embrace the joy and fulfillment that comes from nurturing your body and mind through fitness. Let your exercise routine be a source of strength, a testament to your dedication, and a reflection of your commitment to your own lifelong well-being.

THANKS FOR READING

Dear reader,

Thank you for reading *Daily Exercise Integration: Dynamic Fitness Routines, Exercise Recovery Methods, and More.*

If you enjoyed this book, please leave a review where you bought it. It helps more than most people think.

Get the EXERCISE ESSENTIALS Bundle For FREE!

www.FunctionalHealth.Coach/Exercise-Essentials-Bundle

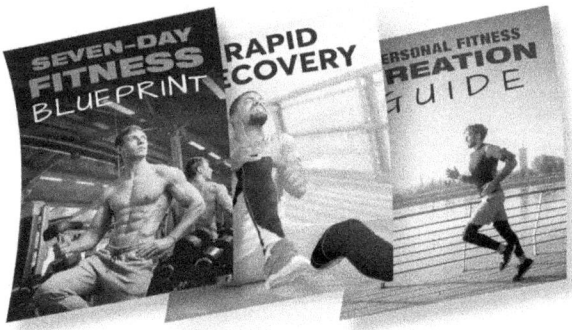

Includes:

- Personal Fitness Creation Guide
- Seven-Day Fitness Blueprint
- Rapid Recovery

Get them all FREE here: www.FunctionalHealth.Coach/Exercise-Essentials-Bundle

ABOUT SAM FURY

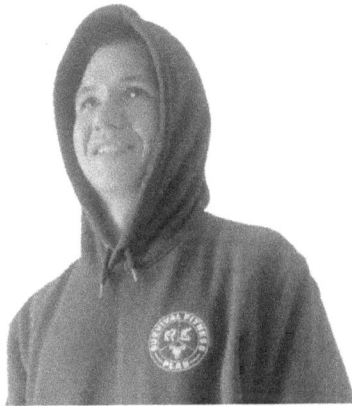

Health Coach - Content Creator - Optimist

www.SamFury.com

amazon.com/author/samfury

goodreads.com/SamFury

facebook.com/SamFuryOfficial

instagram.com/samfuryofficial

youtube.com/@FunctionalHealthShow

REFERENCES

https://acefitness.org

https://acsm.org

https://amazon.com

https://amtamassage.org

https://apa.org

https://bodybuilding.com

https://doi.org

https://harpercollins.com

https://health.clevelandclinic.org

https://health.harvard.edu

https://healthline.com

https://heart.org

https://journals.humankinetics.com

https://journals.lww.com

https://journals.plos.org

https://journals.sagepub.com

https://livestrong.com

https://mayoclinic.org

https://ncbi.nlm.nih.gov

https://ncbtmb.org

https://nccih.nih.gov

https://niams.nih.gov

https://ods.od.nih.gov

https://onlinelibrary.wiley.com

https://open.edu

https://psycnet.apa.org

https://pubmed.ncbi.nlm.nih.gov

https://researchgate.net

https://sciepub.com

https://scirp.org

https://simonandschuster.com

https://sma.org

https://us.humankinetics.com

https://wiley.com/